No Gym Needed

The Beginners Guide To
Easy At-Home, Low-Impact Workouts

LISE CARTWRIGHT

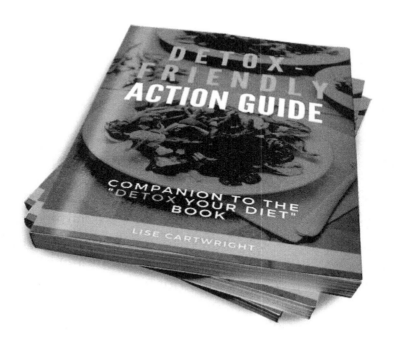

As a HUGE thank you for taking a chance on me (and yourself!) and grabbing this book, I'd love to give you the **_Detox Your Diet Action Guide_**.

It's full of helpful tips & tricks to help you get your diet on track so that you can maximize your health and wellness results from all angles.

Grab it here >> https:// www.hustleandgroove.com/dydguide

Dedication

You. Yes you, my dear reader. This book is dedicated to you.

To the you that is sick of trying to do exercises that don't work for you, to the you that is tired of not moving.

To the you that is ready to make a healthy change!

You got this :-)

Table of Contents

INTRODUCTION

The Challenge

Breaking Down the Barriers to Getting Fit and Healthy

So many readers of my first book in this series have asked for this book: *No Gym Needed: The Beginners Guide to Quick & Easy, At-Home, Low-Impact, Body-Weight Exercises.*

In the first book, *No Gym Needed: Quick & Simple Workouts for Gals on the Go*, I provide an at-home solution that assumes you've already exercised in the past.

You know what different exercises are and you're relatively experienced.

This book, in comparison, is for people who are struggling with any type of exercising at all, whether due to an ongoing injury or an issue with weight.

I felt it was time that those that are struggling — you — had access to a book and a plan that suited you and your exercise level.

It doesn't matter what your situation is, exercising is an important part of feeling good. It helps keep your bones and muscles supple and keeps your major organs working, allowing you to lead a happier and healthier life.

This book was developed to help you to fit in exercises and routines that provide you with the results you want, in a succinct and easy-to-read manner.

This book is for women who suffer from ongoing injuries, are overweight and have a general lack of motivation to hit the gym or exercise in general.

As a full-time freelancer, entrepreneur, and previous 9-5er, I've mastered the art of figuring out how to fit exercise into my days and look after myself, without owning a gym membership or any special types of equipment.

I've read and tested hundreds of different weight loss workouts and healthy lifestyle options to achieve a body and lifestyle I'm happy with.

This book is designed to get you moving again. But, it's only a book. The moving part; you gotta take care of that yourself. In other words, you have to take action. You have to do the exercises.

If you don't do the exercises, nothing will change. It's as simple as that.

The ideas, routines and workouts presented in this book can be implemented and actioned by anyone, anywhere, and they will provide you with ways to start exercising and feeling healthy today.

"We are what we repeatedly do". ~ Aristotle

No Gym Needed: The Beginners Guide provides you with clear and actionable steps to get you on the path to regular exercise and ultimately, a better, healthier you.

The ideas, routines and lifestyle hacks you're about to read have been proven to create life-changing and long-lasting results. All you have to do to achieve a healthier, fitter you is to keep reading.

Each chapter will provide insights as you strive to start exercising and taking care of your health.

Take control of your body right now. Make it work for you and create a body you love, from the outside in.

You'll learn how to change exercises you see and want to give a try, plus you'll also be provided with exercises and routines you CAN do now.

For now, sit back, get comfy and get ready to learn about the solution I've developed to solve the issue of fitting exercise into your life without needing to join a gym.

We'll discuss some lifestyle hacks here as well. Read on to better understand the solutions and learn how you should get started.

CHAPTER 1: YOUR SOLUTION

What I Discovered

As I researched and tried different routines and ideas, I started seeing that there were some core exercises that could be used to design the body I wanted. There were also some lifestyle hacks I could apply to my day, so that I could fit in exercise.

I've also worked with woman who have injuries, severe health issues like diabetes, or are overweight and just unable to exercise at the gym.

Part of this process included discovering that I didn't need to belong to a gym, nor did I need to exercise for hours at a time to achieve the results I wanted — a body that I WAS HAPPY with.

That last little sentence is important. Before you begin any form of exercising, you need to determine why or who you're doing this for.

You need to realize that you should only be doing this for yourself.

You'll find routines that take less than 30 minutes to complete — because who wants to spend their life exercising? Not me.

The main point of this book is help you get back into a

regular, consistent exercise routine. You'll use exercises that you can do, without injuring yourself further, or feeling like you can't do them.

The best way to take advantage of this book is to do the exercises. If you find them difficult, try the suggested modifications.

Remember "Can or do not, there is no try" ~ Yoda

What's Required From You
Along the way, you're going to need to decide if you want to be healthy and fit. Which I'm assuming you do, otherwise why are you reading this book?

Part of the process of fitting exercise into your day is about developing habits. You'll get plenty of help and advice from this book about how to do this. How to exercise quickly while still getting the results you're after.

A large part of losing weight or designing the body you want relies on understanding the changes in your body. This is why we need to track and measure our progress.

Don't worry; you don't have to weigh yourself if you don't want to. It's not necessary to track and measure your actual weight. Instead, we'll focus on taking more meaningful measurements, such as your upper-thigh measurement or your hip and waist measurements. What are we measuring when we do this? Body fat. This is a much better indicator of weight loss and body design than what the scales say.

We'll cover this in more detail in Chapter 5.

By measuring parts of your body, you can see where fat is replaced with muscle. It's a far better motivator when you see centimetres (or inches) melting away than jumping on scales that tell you that you haven't lost any weight.

After 30 days of consistent, regular exercise, your fitness level will have improved, and that will be evident through the tracking and measuring you'll be doing.

While there are a few fitness tracking apps available (which I'll mention later in this book), I've found that writing everything down in a little journal works best. There's something about putting pen to paper that makes your progress that much sweeter.

A Note About Routines
The exercises and routines you'll see in this book are specifically designed for beginners. But if you struggle to do any of the exercises, look for the "modification" option so that no matter what your current situation, you can at least attempt to do an exercise.

This book only includes body-weight exercises or exercises using household weights.

So don't worry — you don't have to run out and buy any special equipment!

What to Expect

This how-to guide is full of easy, accessible exercises based on utilizing your body weight.

Before you start any exercise program, you should seek the advice of your doctor. This is to make sure that what is you're looking to start is going to be safe for you.

Are you ready to get started?!

In the next section we're going to make sure that you've got the right form when exercising. Without correct form, you could injure yourself, target the wrong muscles or injure someone else.

We'll also look at safety while you're exercising, as this is something else you need to factor into your exercise habits.

Lastly, we'll start ***The Beginners No Gym Needed Plan.***

Let's get started!

CHAPTER 2: FORM & SAFETY

Be Aware

Remember, before you start any form of exercise, it's important that you think about the types of exercises you'll be doing.

And that you understand how they should be executed, and where you plan to do them.

If you don't have the correct form, you could end up injuring yourself or those around you.

If you're not aware of your surroundings, or don't let others know what your exercise plans are, you could find yourself in some icky situations too.

Read on to avoid any negative outcomes that prevent you from achieving your exercise goals.

Form

Before you start your workouts, you need to make sure that you understand how to protect yourself from injuries. Learning the correct way to do an exercise, or the correct "form" for each exercise is important to your own safety and results.

If you don't learn how to do an exercise the right way, you could end up damaging your back or muscles or worse, breaking a bone.

No one wants to end up with a "stuffed" back because they didn't take the time to read and learn how to execute a specific exercise. Make sure you check your form by watching yourself in a mirror as you do each exercise and by following the steps below.

Each routine in this book provides you with specific instructions on how to do each move, but if you want to make sure your form is correct (which you should), then this is what you need to know.

Upper and Lower Body Exercises
Follow these steps to ensure that you're protecting yourself from injury:

1. If using weights (optional — none of the exercises within this book use weights), never jerk the weight behind you or above your head. You want to aim for a fluid, deliberate motion. Also, make sure that you've got a good grip on them, particularly if you're doing squats and have the weights resting on your thighs or shoulders. Make sure the weights are secure before you begin the exercise.
2. When working on your back or core muscles, always make sure that your core is pulled in tight. This means pulling your belly button into your back — basically sucking your tummy in. You need to keep it that way the whole time you're working on your back or core area. This prevents lower back injury and pulled abdominal

muscles.

3. Never fully extend your arms, and keep your elbows soft, particularly when you're using weights of any kind (household items included). If you fully extend and lock your elbows in place, you risk injuring your biceps, triceps, and elbow joints. Also, when doing lunges or squats, never lock your knees in place as you're coming up; always keep them soft. This protects your knees and keeps the muscles you're targeting engaged and working.

4. When working on any part of your upper or lower body, keep your stance soft. This means keeping your knees slightly bent and your weight pushing through your heels. This will help keep you balanced and takes some of the pressure off your upper body.

Exercise Hack

No matter what exercise you're doing, always suck your belly button into your lower back. This ensures that you're protecting your lower back at all times and helps prevent injuries developing. It also provides a bonus workout for your core!

Safety Best Practices

While the above is focused on form and execution, this area is focused on making sure you're safe while you work out, particularly if you're working out alone or outdoors.

This is where planning and scheduling your exercise is

key. You need to think about where you're going to exercise ahead of time so that you can ensure your own safety.

Some things to consider as you're exercising:

1. If you're working out alone, make sure that someone knows what you're doing, particularly if you're using weights of any kind. This is especially true if you work from home and no one will be home to see you until after 5pm. The easiest way for me to do this is to check in with my husband at lunchtime. That way, if he doesn't hear from me, he knows something's up — you should implement something similar.

2. If you're planning to workout outside, let someone know where you'll be, particularly if you're going for a run and have your headphones in or you're working out at a park in the middle of the day. Make sure you are aware of your surroundings and of anyone else around you.

3. Be smart about getting started. Take it easy initially and then progressively increase the difficulty of the exercises you're doing. If you feel something pull or twinge while exercise, stop. Stretch the area where you feel the pain and then try again. Take it easy and rest if you need to. I fractured my ankle running and ignored the pain and continued to exercise on it for days afterwards. Luckily I didn't do any permanent damage, but it meant I had to rest for 6 weeks with no exercise!

There's no harm in being smart and being aware. If you work out by yourself, always let someone know what you're up to, even if it's a quick post on Facebook or quick snap of where you are on Instagram.

Be smart, be aware, be safe.

Stretching

At the end of each exercise routine you complete, you need to stretch, even if you've only got a couple of minutes. If you don't, you'll feel it and be too sore to exercise for a few days.

I remember a program that I started a few years ago called the "butt, thigh and leg workout" that was all about targeting those three main areas using a weighted belt.

The first few days were hard, but I loved the feeling of working out my butt and thighs — problem areas for me because I'm pear-shaped.

Anyway, on the third day, I literally could not walk. Picture this if you can (and I'm sure you will!):

I was living in a 2-story townhouse and my bedroom was upstairs. I went up to bed on day 2, and by day 3 I couldn't even walk, let alone face walking down a flight of stairs. What did I do instead?

I had to sit down at the top and butt-scoot down a flight of 20 stairs (much to the delight of my roommates at the time). I don't know what was worse, the pain or the embarrassment!

Had I taken the time to stretch my muscles on days 1 and 2, I would have been sore on day 3 still, but it's unlikely a flight of stairs would have kicked my ass. Lesson learned.

So, if you want to avoid doing the "butt walk of shame", you need to make time to stretch.

In case you need more reasons, here are five benefits you'll get from stretching, besides avoiding injury:

1. **Circulation**
    Your muscles work hard when you're working out, so hard that blood circulation can slow down, preventing nutrients reaching your muscles. This is a large part of why your muscles hurt the next day, and why you should stretch. By stretching, you increase blood flow and the nutrients can then be supplied to your muscles when they need them most. This reduces soreness and allows you to exercise those same muscles the following day.

2. **Flexibility**
    This is just common sense. The more flexible you are, the easier exercising becomes and the less strain there is on major areas of your body. As you get older, your muscles become shorter and

tighter, so the more you stretch, the more you lengthen those muscles and the longer they'll be able to support you.

3. **Joint Motion**

    By stretching, you increase your level of flexibility, which leads to an increase in motion for your joints. It's win-win as far as I can see. Range of motion becomes important the older you get, so do yourself a favour and stretch whenever you work out to ensure that you have the use of your muscles for many, many years to come.

4. **Stress Reduction**

    Along with exercising, stretching also helps to reduce stress, not just on your mind, but also on your body. By stretching, you release the tension in your muscles, not just from working out, but also from the stress of the day. You'll also release endorphins, just like you do while exercising, which will help to improve your mood and the way you feel overall.

5. **Reduce Lower Back Pain**

    Stretching also helps to relieve tension you have built up in your lower back during an exercise session. Chronic lower back pain is one of the most common ailments that people deal with, so stretching this area will help relieve the pain and help strengthen back muscles as well.

Now that you understand just how important it is, make

sure you refer to the resources page for the list of the top 10 stretches you should do following each workout.

Now that we've covered form and stretching, the next section is where the fun really begins! It's time to dive headfirst into your **No Gym Needed plan**.

CHAPTER 3: THE BEGINNERS "NO GYM NEEDED" PLAN

The Plan Explained

Welcome to the *Beginners No Gym Needed Plan*. This chapter focuses on helping you get into a regular exercise program to increase your fitness, help you feel healthy and ultimately, manage your weight.

As you have already experienced, losing weight can be tough when you're already carrying more weight than you want... Standard exercise routines and gym programs don't take into account your unique circumstances, which is super frustrating.

This chapter is all about helping you get moving again. If you can't do an exercise, see the suggestions to modify it. Remember, the goal is to get you moving. Focus on that rather than trying to lose weight first.

You'll feel less frustrated if you focus on movement first. Losing weight takes time and is not just based on your exercise routine. It takes a holistic view, with the foods that you eat playing a much larger role in your weight management than exercise.

Everything you see in this book will help you move and increase your fitness. But to reach your weight loss goals, you'll need to also be looking at what you're eating too.

The routines in this book are split into two different sections:

1. Body-weight Routines
2. Weighted Routines (using household items or dumbbells)

The aim is to choose the exercises and routines that work best for you right now. If you find any of the exercises or routines difficult to do or complete, read the modification suggestions to make the exercises easier.

A couple of things to remember before you begin ANY exercise regime:

- Check with your doctor to make sure that what you're planning to do is right for you and your situation
- It pays to exercise on a near-empty stomach. If you must eat, eat something like a banana or other piece of fruit and wait 15 minutes before you start exercising.
- Don't drink your calories! Have water on hand while you exercise, but don't get the flavored water. If you need flavor, add in a slice of lemon or lime instead.
- Listen to your body. If you feel shooting pain, stop what you're doing. You can expect exercises to feel hard or your body to be stiff initially, but this is normal and will ease the more you do the

exercises.

Always have healthy snacks available. In your bag, on your desk, in the car, around your house – just have them on hand. What's healthy? Protein powder or meal replacement powder + water, nuts and seeds, baby carrots, etc. Fuel your body with the right foods and it will take care of the rest.

If you want to really look at your diet, check out my other book, **Detox Your Diet**: *A 28-Day Detox Plan — How to Banish Addictive Foods, Lose Weight Naturally & Send Your Energy Levels Through the Roof!*

Visit https://www.detoxyourdietplan.com/the-book/ to get your own copy.

Being Consistent With Exercising
When it comes to how often you should exercise when you're getting started, there are a couple of points to keep in mind:

- If you're exercising with any type of weights, you need to allow 1-2 days of rest between weighted exercises to allow muscles to repair themselves. Keep this in mind when you're using any of the weighted exercise routines.
- With cardio exercises, you can do these more frequently, up to 3-5 times per week. These are perfect to do on your non-weight days.

Ready? Let's get started! Read on to learn about your

first beginners workout routine!

Go-To Exercises

Before we get stuck into different beginner routines, you need to be familiar with the different exercises we're going to be using to make up these routines.

Study the exercises below and make sure you're comfortable doing them.

You can see videos for each exercise on the Resources Page here:

https://www.hustleandgroove.com/ngnbresources

Password: ngnb@2717

Ready? Get started now.

#1: Squats

- Beginner: 20 reps [with weights use milk bottle option x 3 sets]
- Intermediate: 45 reps [with weights use sand-filled coffee canisters x 3 sets]
- Advanced: 60 reps [with weights use 5-10 lbs bag of potatoes x 3 sets]

Repeat the exercise 3 times.

Refer to the image below to see how to do this exercise with correct form.

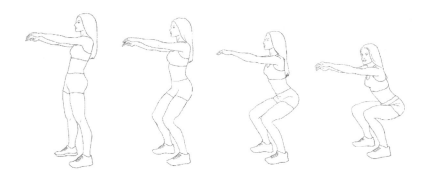

How-to:
When doing this exercise, you want to keep your weight in your heels, pushing down through your heels when you squat and then also pushing up through your heels when you stand (if performing an assisted squat).

Do not over-extend your knees or lock them in place on your way up. Instead, keep knees soft and don't straighten them on your way up. This will keep your upper leg muscles engaged at all times.

1. Start with your feet shoulder-width apart, with your toes slightly pointing outwards.
2. Pull your belly into your back, so that you've got proper support.
3. Lower your bum to the floor, stopping about halfway down. This action should be like you were about to sit in a chair, so stick your bum out but keep your chest and head level.

MODIFICATIONS

If you're just getting started and aren't familiar with this exercise or you don't feel you can hold your weight on your own, you might find it helpful to use a chair to help you with this exercise.

Pretend you're going to sit on the chair and hover just above it when you feel the back of your thighs grazing the chair (think hamstrings). Or, if you feel like that is still going to be difficult, use the chair to balance yourself by placing the chair on one side of your body and holding onto it as you lower yourself down.

Remember, you don't have to do a deep squat to begin with.

Alternative Exercise: If you're not able to do a squat at all, you could do a Glute Bridge, where you lie on your back on the ground, with your feet flat on the floor, knees up as if you were going to do a sit up.

Pushing through your feet, lift your bum off the ground as high as you can go, and squeeze your butt muscles. Hold this for 3 seconds and lower.

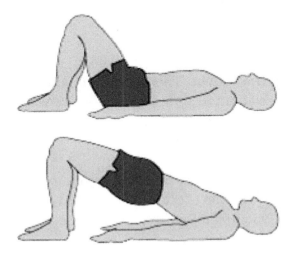

Repeat 10-20 times.

#2: Mountain Climbers

- Beginner: 10 reps
- Intermediate: 35 reps
- Advanced: 50 reps

Refer to the image below to see how to do this exercise with the correct form.

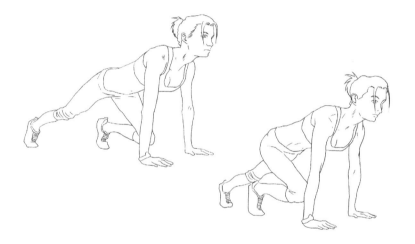

The key to doing this exercise right is to keep your upper body tight, tummy muscles pulled in, and pushing all your weight through your legs.

How-to:
1. Start with your feet slightly shoulder-width apart, with toes slightly   pointing outwards.
2. Lower your body straight down, keeping all the weight in the back of your heels.
3. Place your hands on the ground in front of you

and pulling your tummy into your back, kick your feet backwards, landing on your toes.

4. Pull one leg in towards your waist, keep the other leg out straight.

5. Pretend you're walking up a mountain, jump-changing between each   stride as you change legs.

MODIFICATIONS

There are several ways you can modify the mountain climber to suit your current situation.

#1: Use a chair to support your arms by placing them on the seat part of the chair. This allows you to be semi-upright as you do the mountain climbers.

#2: If the chair option is still difficult, stand up normally and use the back of the chair to support you as you raise your knees towards your chest as if you were climbing really high stairs. Start slow and the slowing increase your pace.

#3: Rather than "walking up a mountain" for your mountain climbers, try pulling your knee to the opposite elbow, like you might if you were doing bicycle crunches. This makes the exercise easier to complete.

All of these options offer varying degrees of difficulty. Choose the one that best suits your current situation.

#3: Jumping Jacks

- Beginner: 30 seconds
- Intermediate: 60 seconds
- Advanced: 120 seconds

Repeat 2 times.

Refer to the image below to see how to do this exercise with the correct form.

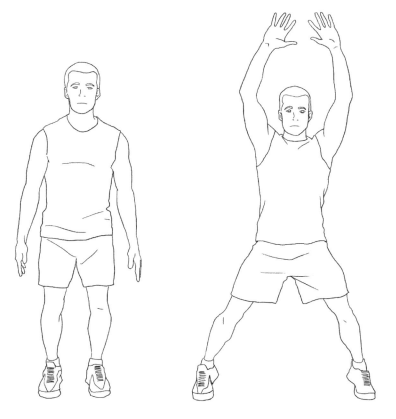

How-to:
The key to doing this exercise properly is making sure that your hands clap above your head and that your feet are slightly pointed outwards. Do the movement as fast as you can in the time you've chosen, depending on your level.

You can add weights to this exercise by adding sand or pebbles to a pair of old socks and holding on to them or tying them to a belt; the more socks you hold, the harder it will be.

MODIFICATIONS
Jumping Jacks are a cardio-based exercise and are great for lifting your heart-rate.

But they can also be hard on your knees. If you find a standard jumping jack difficult to do, follow these options instead.

#1: Rather than jumping, step side to side instead. You can do this as fast or as slow as you wish. One repetition is a step each side. Still raise your arms, but instead of raising them out to the side, simply raise them straight up.

#2: If you find raising your arms too hard, lift them halfway instead and slowly increase how high your raise them every time you do jumping jacks.

Alternative Exercise: Instead of doing a full jumping jack, replace the exercise by marching in place. You can march as fast or as slow as you like. Make sure to swing your arms as well, to get the most out of this easier option.

#4: Plank

- Beginner: 20 seconds
- Intermediate: 45 seconds
- Advanced: 60 seconds

Refer to the image below to see how to do this exercise with the correct form.

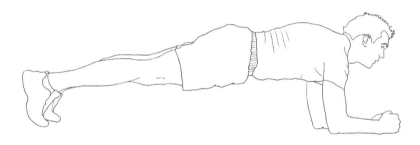

The Plank is a great workout for your core. If you can do this every day, either as part of your exercise routine or just when you're watching TV, you'll start to see a difference in 30 days.

How-to:
1. Lay down on your tummy.
2. Prop yourself up on your elbows, shoulders tight and arms strong.
3. Pull your tummy into your back and lift your

body up, resting on your toes.

4. Keep your back flat and hold this stance for your chosen amount of time.

MODIFICATIONS

You can decrease the difficulty of this exercise by propping yourself up on your hands rather than your elbows.

You can also use a chair to balance yourself on too, as long as you're pulling your tummy tight and keeping your arms straight, you will still see the benefits of this exercise.

#5: Push-ups

- Beginner: 10 reps
- Intermediate: 40 reps
- Advanced: 60 reps

Repeat 2 times.

Refer to the image below to see how to do this exercise with the correct form.

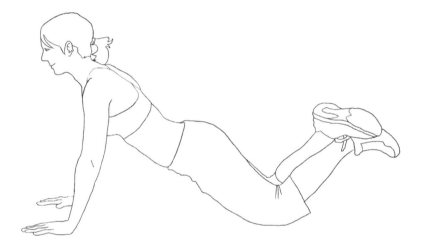

MODIFICATIONS

As a beginner, you should start on your knees; as an intermediate, on your knees but with your torso elongated (as shown in the picture); and advanced should be a full push-up off the toes.

The closer your knees are to your chest, the easier it is

to do. As long as you keep a strong form through your shoulders and arms, you will see results from the easiest option.

#6: Lunges

- Beginners: 5 reps each leg
- Intermediate: 15 reps each leg
- Advanced: 25 reps each leg

Repeat 2 times.

Refer to the image below to see how to do this exercise with the correct form.

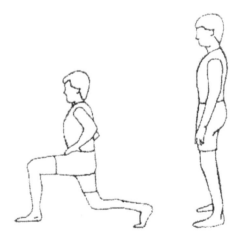

How-to:
1. Start with your feet shoulder width apart. Place your hands on your hips and take a big step forward with your right foot.

2. All of the weight should be on the foot that is stepped forward, with your back leg used to keep you balanced.

3. Push off on the foot that is forward and step back. Repeat on the other leg.

MODIFICATIONS

If you find taking a big step forward difficult, just take a normal step forward and lower your body down half-way.

If you find a forward lunge like this difficult to do, period, try a side lunge instead. Step out to the left as wide as you can go and then step back. Repeat on the other side.

You can also use a chair to help you balance as well as take some of your weight.

Lunges are an important exercise as they increase your flexibility, so try and do one of the modified versions if you can.

Refer to the Resources Page here: https://www.hustleandgroove.com/ngnbresources — for videos on how to do these exercises.

Don't forget, you need this password to access the resources page: *ngnb@2717*

Next, we're going to jump into some body weight routines using a combination of these exercises.

Remember, if you struggle with any of the exercises, refer to the modifications above to make it easer.

Body Weight Routines

To ease yourself into a regular exercise routine, I want to start you off with body weight routines using the exercises we covered in the last section.

This allows you to get used to exercising and used to the types of exercises you can and should be doing.

To avoid injury, and if you're unsure about what is best for you, seek the advice of your medical practitioner.

Always start off with the easiest version of an exercise and don't push yourself too hard in the first few weeks.

Once you've been exercising, you can start to increase repetitions and focus on your form and how you can push yourself more.

Below you'll find a 14-day and 30-day workout chart that you can use to get started with.

> *Want a portable version of these workouts? Check the Resources Page and you'll find downloadable PDF versions of all the workout routines for your convenience!*

None of these routines need weights, so they are ideal for beginners or if you're traveling.

14-Day Workout: Kick-Starting Your Exercise Habit

Use this if you haven't been exercising for a while, have an injury or are getting started and need to ease yourself back into exercising and setting up regular routines:

Day 1	Warm up by marching in place, making sure to swing your arms high • Walk for 20 minutes at a moderate pace • Squats x 20 (repeat twice) • Plank for 20 seconds off your hands (not elbows)
Day 2	REST
Day 3	Warm up by marching in place, making sure to swing your arms high • Walk for 20 minutes at a moderate pace • Jumping Jacks for 30 seconds (repeat twice) • Push ups x 10 reps (repeat twice)
Day 4	REST
Day 5	Warm up by marching in place, making sure to swing your arms high • Walk for 20 minutes at a moderate pace • Squats x 20 (repeat twice) • Plank for 20 seconds off your hands (not elbows)
Day 6	REST

Day 7	Warm up by marching in place, making sure to swing your arms high • Walk for 20 minutes at a moderate pace • Jumping Jacks for 30 seconds (repeat twice) • Push ups x 10 reps (repeat twice)
Day 8	REST
Day 9	Warm up by marching in place, making sure to swing your arms high • Walk for 20 minutes at a moderate pace • Lunges x 5 each leg (repeat twice) • Mountain climbers x 10 reps
Day 10	REST
Day 11	Warm up by marching in place, making sure to swing your arms high • Walk for 20 minutes at a moderate pace • Push-ups x 10 reps (repeat twice) • Jumping Jacks for 30 seconds (repeat twice)
Day 12	REST
Day 13	Warm up by marching in place, making sure to swing your arms high • Walk for 20 minutes at a moderate pace • Lunges x 5 each leg (repeat twice) • Mountain climbers x 10 reps
Day 14	REST

30-Day Workout: Creating the Exercise Habit

Move onto this 30-Day Workout once you've completed the first 14-days above.

Continue with this routine for 3 months, reviewing every 30 days to see whether you need to make any changes, such as increasing reps or making modifications, or whether you're ready to head to the next section, which is all about adding weights to your exercises to strengthen your muscles.

Day 1	Warm up by marching in place, making sure to swing your arms high • Walk for 30 minutes at a moderate pace • Squats x 25 (repeat twice) • Plank for 40 seconds off your hands (noT elbows)
Day 2	REST
Day 3	Warm up by marching in place, making sure to swing your arms high • Walk for 30 minutes at a moderate pace • Jumping Jacks for 30 seconds (repeat twice) • Push ups x 10 reps (repeat twice)
Day 4	REST

Day 5	Warm up by marching in place, making sure to swing your arms high • Walk for 30 minutes at a moderate pace • Squats x 25 (repeat twice) • Plank for 40 seconds off your hands (not elbows)
Day 6	REST
Day 7	Warm up by marching in place, making sure to swing your arms high • Walk for 30 minutes at a moderate pace • Jumping Jacks for 30 seconds (repeat twice) • Push ups x 10 reps (repeat twice)
Day 8	REST
Day 9	Warm up by marching in place, making sure to swing your arms high • Walk for 30 minutes at a moderate pace • Lunges x 5 each leg (repeat twice) • Mountain climbers x 15 reps
Day 10	REST
Day 11	Warm up by marching in place, making sure to swing your arms high • Walk for 30 minutes at a moderate pace • Push-ups x 10 reps (repeat twice) • Jumping Jacks for 30 seconds (repeat twice)
Day 12	REST

Day 13	Warm up by marching in place, making sure to swing your arms high • Walk for 30 minutes at a moderate pace • Lunges x 5 each leg (repeat twice) • Mountain climbers x 15 reps
Day 14	REST
Day 15	Warm up by marching in place, making sure to swing your arms high • Walk for 30 minutes at a moderate pace • Squats x 25 (repeat twice) • Plank for 40 seconds off your elbows
Day 16	REST
Day 17	Warm up by marching in place, making sure to swing your arms high • Walk for 30 minutes at a moderate pace • Lunges x 5 each leg (repeat twice) • Mountain climbers x 15 reps
Day 18	REST
Day 19	Warm up by marching in place, making sure to swing your arms high • Walk for 30 minutes at a moderate pace • Squats x 25 (repeat twice) • Plank for 40 seconds off your elbows
Day 20	REST

Day 21	Warm up by marching in place, making sure to swing your arms high • Walk for 30 minutes at a moderate pace • Lunges x 5 each leg (repeat twice) • Mountain climbers x 15 reps
Day 22	REST
Day 23	Warm up by marching in place, making sure to swing your arms high • Walk for 30 minutes at a moderate pace • Jumping Jacks for 30 seconds (repeat twice) • Push ups x 15 reps (repeat twice)
Day 24	REST
Day 25	Warm up by marching in place, making sure to swing your arms high • Walk for 30 minutes at a moderate pace • Squats x 25 (repeat twice) • Plank for 40 seconds off your elbows
Day 26	REST
Day 27	Warm up by marching in place, making sure to swing your arms high • Walk for 30 minutes at a moderate pace • Jumping Jacks for 30 seconds (repeat twice) • Push ups x 15 reps (repeat twice)
Day 28	REST

Day 29	Warm up by marching in place, making sure to swing your arms high • Walk for 30 minutes at a moderate pace • Squats x 25 (repeat twice) • Plank for 40 seconds off your elbows
Day 30	REST

Exercise Hacks

Hack 1 - If you want to reduce your blood pressure and increase your deep sleep cycles, exercise in the morning, before 11am.

A study conducted by Appalachian State University (www.news.appstate.edu/2011/06/13/early-morning-exercise/) found that people who exercised in the mornings spent up to 75% more time in reparative "deep sleep" than those who exercised later in the day.

Hack 2 - Look at adding intermittent fasting to your diet (www.lifehack.org/articles/lifestyle/intermittent-fasting-the-ultimate-weight-loss-hack.html) . This post from Nerd Fitness goes into all the nerdy details.

Studies show that you can lose 2-3 pounds (0.9 - 1.3 kilograms) per week through fasting. Start with fasting for 12 hours each day and work your way up to 16-20 hours (with 20 hours being the maximum time to fast) per day. This is a great way to burn excess body fat quickly and safely. Make sure you check out this diet properly before starting it!

Hack 3 - Eat less than 75 grams of carbs per day while you're looking to lose weight. 75 grams is equal to 1.5 cups of rice, 2 slices of bread or 18 ounces of cola.

Doing this one thing can help you to lose up to 3 pounds (1.3 kg) per week plus whatever you lose working out.

In the next section, we're going to switch to weighted routines. You'll find options for body weight and weights (using household items), so choose the options that work for you.

Turn the page to learn about my special "No Gym Needed" weighted routines.

Weighted Routines

Strength training is a great way to improve your fitness and help with weight loss. The healthier your muscles are, the faster they'll burn off fat.

I recommend using weights after at least 30 days of body weight routines so that you're body is used to exercising and has a bit of muscle memory built up.

You need to make sure you're careful when using weights as well, as you don't want to hurt yourself.

If you've never used weights before and are worried about hurting yourself, follow these steps.

#1:Take it slow
#2: Refer back to the form chapter (Chapter 2)
#3: And if you do feel any pain, see your doctor immediately

Always start off light and don't push yourself too hard in the first few days of starting on weights.

> *If you can't complete the reps in the amount of sets stipulated, then the weight you're using is too heavy. Make sure you switch to a lighter weight and work your way up slowly.*
> *The reps and sets should be challenging, but not impossible.*

Below you'll find a 14-day and 30-day workout chart similar to what you've just completed in the body weight routine section.

All of these routines require weights from around the home, and are designed to build upon the body weight routines from the previous section. If you find it difficult to do the lightest weight, stop using weights and continue with just the body weight routines.

I'd recommend that you complete at least 3 months of body weight routines before introducing weights, particularly if you've got any ongoing injuries.

Remember, speak to your doctor before you begin ANY exercise routine to make sure that you are doing what is right for your situation.

Some suggested options for your "No Gym Needed" weights:

- 2 x 2 or 3-litre milk bottles
- 5-10 lbs bag of potatoes (2-4 kg)
- 2-3 heavy, hardcover books
- 2 x cans of soup or any liquid-in-a-can
- 2 x coffee considers (fill with sand for heavier weights)
- 2 x water bottles (1-litre or more)
- 2 x bulk items like rice or beans - 5-10 lbs (2-4 kg)
- Your kids!

If you want to buy weights (remember, they are NOT required to do these exercises), these are some suggestions:

- Dumbbells
- Kettle bells

Some suggested weight sizes for dumbbells or kettle bells:

- 3 sets of dumbbells (weight will depend on your level)
    - Beginner: start with smaller weights – 4.4 lbs (2 x 2kg), 11 lbs (2 x 5kg) and 22 lbs (2 x 10kg)
    - Intermediate: start with 11 lbs (2 x 5kg), 22 lbs (2 x 10kg) and 33 lbs (2 x 15kg)
    - Advanced: start with 44 lbs (2 x 20kg), 66 lbs (2 x 30kg) and 110 lbs (2 x 50kg)

- 2 kettle bells (weight will depend on your level)
    - Beginner: start with 17.5 lbs (1 x 8kg) and 26.4 lbs (1 x 12kg)
    - Intermediate: start with 26.4 lbs (1 x 12kg) and 35.2 lbs (1 x 16kg)
    - Advanced: start with 35.2 lbs (1 x 16kg) and 57.3 lbs (1 x 26kg)

It's not always about how much weight you're lifting; it's about correct form and the amount of sets you do. Keep this in mind when deciding on what weight options you choose.

It's important that initially you start out with the body weight routines and slowly introduce these weight options, particularly if you haven't exercised for a while or have an injury.

Weighted Hacks

Hack 1 - Instead of dumbbells, you can use 1-litre, 1.5-litre and 2-litre bottles. Where possible, make sure they are filled with water. You don't want a bottle of Coke bursting on you mid-workout. Believe me, it's not pretty!

Hack 2 - Instead of kettle bells, you can use bags of sugar, rice, flour, etc., anything that you can purchase in bulk and that weighs more than 2.2 lbs (1kg).

14-Day Workout: Introducing Weighted Exercises

Use this to ease yourself into using weights, always starting off at the lightest weight and work your way up.

Day 1	Warm up by marching in place, making sure to swing your arms high
	• Walk/Jog for 30 minutes at a moderate pace
	• 20 Squats - repeat twice with your choice of weight (resting either on your shoulders or in your hands)
	• Plank for 60 seconds off your elbows
Day 2	REST

Day 3	Warm up by marching in place, making sure to swing your arms high ■ Walk/Jog for 30 minutes at a moderate pace ■ Jumping Jacks for 60 seconds (repeat twice) ■ Push ups x 15 reps (repeat twice)
Day 4	REST
Day 5	Warm up by marching in place, making sure to swing your arms high ■ Walk for 30 minutes at a moderate pace ■ 20 Squats - repeat twice with your choice of weight ■ Plank for 60 seconds off your elbows
Day 6	REST
Day 7	Warm up by marching in place, making sure to swing your arms high ■ Walk for 30 minutes at a moderate pace ■ Jumping Jacks for 60 seconds (repeat twice) ■ Push ups x 15 reps (repeat twice)
Day 8	REST

Day 9	Warm up by marching in place, making sure to swing your arms high ■ Walk/Jog for 30 minutes at a moderate pace ■ Lunges x 10 each leg - repeat twice using your choice of weight (holding in your hands or resting on your shoulders) ■ Mountain climbers x 20 reps (repeat twice)
Day 10	REST
Day 11	Warm up by marching in place, making sure to swing your arms high ■ Walk/Jog for 30 minutes at a moderate pace ■ Push-ups x 15 reps (repeat twice) ■ Jumping Jacks for 30 seconds (repeat twice)
Day 12	REST
Day 13	Warm up by marching in place, making sure to swing your arms high ■ Walk/Jog for 30 minutes at a moderate pace ■ Lunges x 10 each leg - repeat twice using your choice of weight ■ Mountain climbers x 20 reps (repeat twice)
Day 14	REST

30-Day Workout: Using Weights Regularly

Move onto this workout once you've completed the first 14 days. Review and decide if you need to change your weights or stick with what you currently have. Repeat this workout for 3 months, making sure to review every 30 days.

Day 1	Warm up by marching in place, making sure to swing your arms high
	▪ Walk/Jog for 30 minutes at a moderate pace
	▪ Lunges x 15 each leg - repeat twice with your choice of weight (try to increase from the last 14 days)
	▪ Mountain climbers x 15 reps (repeat twice)
Day 2	REST
Day 3	Warm up by marching in place, making sure to swing your arms high
	▪ Walk/Jog for 30 minutes at a moderate pace
	▪ Jumping Jacks for 30 seconds (repeat twice)
	▪ Push ups x 20 reps (repeat twice)
Day 4	REST

Day 5	Warm up by marching in place, making sure to swing your arms high • Walk/Jog for 30 minutes at a moderate pace • Lunges x 15 each leg - repeat twice with your choice of weight • Mountain climbers x 15 reps (repeat twice)
Day 6	REST
Day 7	Warm up by marching in place, making sure to swing your arms high • Walk/Jog for 30 minutes at a moderate pace • Jumping Jacks for 30 seconds (repeat twice) • Push ups x 20 reps (repeat twice)
Day 8	REST
Day 9	Warm up by marching in place, making sure to swing your arms high • Walk/Jog for 30 minutes at a moderate pace • 25 Squats - repeat twice with your choice of weight • Push-ups x 20 reps (repeat twice)
Day 10	REST

Day 11	Warm up by marching in place, making sure to swing your arms high ■ Walk/Jog for 30 minutes at a moderate pace ■ Plank for 60 seconds off elbows ■ Lunges x 15 each leg - repeat twice with your choice of weight
Day 12	REST
Day 13	Warm up by marching in place, making sure to swing your arms high ■ Walk/Jog for 30 minutes at a moderate pace ■ 25 Squats - repeat twice with your choice of weight ■ Push-ups x 20 reps (repeat twice)
Day 14	REST
Day 15	Warm up by marching in place, making sure to swing your arms high ■ Walk/Jog for 30 minutes at a moderate pace ■ Plank for 60 seconds off elbows ■ Lunges x 15 each leg - repeat twice with your choice of weight
Day 16	REST

Day 17	Warm up by marching in place, making sure to swing your arms high • Walk/Jog for 30 minutes at a moderate pace • Lunges x 20 each leg - repeat twice with your choice of weight (try to increase from the last 14 days) • Mountain climbers x 25 reps (repeat twice)
Day 18	REST
Day 19	Warm up by marching in place, making sure to swing your arms high • Walk/Jog for 30 minutes at a moderate pace • Jumping Jacks for 60 seconds (repeat twice) • Push ups x 20 reps (repeat three times)
Day 20	REST
Day 21	Warm up by marching in place, making sure to swing your arms high • Walk/Jog for 30 minutes at a moderate pace • Lunges x 20 each leg - repeat twice with your choice of weight (try to increase from the last 14 days) • Mountain climbers x 25 reps (repeat twice)
Day 22	REST

Day 23	Warm up by marching in place, making sure to swing your arms high • Walk/Jog for 30 minutes at a moderate pace • Jumping Jacks for 60 seconds (repeat twice) • Push ups x 20 reps (repeat three times)
Day 24	REST
Day 25	Warm up by marching in place, making sure to swing your arms high • Walk/Jog for 30 minutes at a moderate pace • 35 Squats - repeat twice with your choice of weight • Push-ups x 20 reps (repeat twice)
Day 26	REST
Day 27	Warm up by marching in place, making sure to swing your arms high • Walk/Jog for 30 minutes at a moderate pace • Plank for 60 seconds off elbows • Lunges x 20 each leg - repeat twice with your choice of weight
Day 28	REST

Day 29	Warm up by marching in place, making sure to swing your arms high • Walk/Jog for 30 minutes at a moderate pace • 35 Squats - repeat twice with your choice of weight • Push-ups x 20 reps (repeat twice)
Day 30	REST

Congratulations! If you've stuck to the recommended 30-day routines, you're well on your way to feeling and looking better.

You should have started to see a change in your body, through tightening of your muscles and fat starting to burn off.

But remember, exercising is just a small portion of your weight loss journey.

What you eat contributes to 80% of your weight loss. So if you're exercising 5 times a week but haven't changed your diet, it's likely that you won't have seen the results you want.

Use this book to start your exercising habit and then once you've got this covered, look at your diet and start to make changes there.

In the next chapter, we're going to look at how to track your progress because without tracking what you're doing, it's hard to see the results and changes in your body.

Continue reading to learn more.

CHAPTER 4: TRACK AND MEASURE

Tracking Your Progress

No matter what you do, don't forget to track and measure your progress. This will help you stay focused, as you'll be able to see things progressing.

Keep off the scales as much as possible. They are not your friend. They don't truly reflect weight loss, which is why it's important to measure more than just your weight.

What I have learned is that if I don't track and measure my weight, then I find it far easier to "fall off the wagon".

One of the easiest ways to track your progress is to simply jot down your measurements. I take the measurements of my arms, waist, hips, legs and chest area.

This tells me how many inches I've lost, which relates to body fat. This is a far better indicator of weight-loss progress than what you see on the scales, because muscle is heavier than fat.

I'd also recommend taking a before photo and then one every 30 days, so you can see the changes in your body.

Do yourself a favor and measure your body fat progress instead. It's super rewarding to see inches falling off week after week rather than checking the scales and seeing no change at all.

This is because muscle is heavier than weight. As I said, the scales are not always the best way to measure your progress.

Tracking Your Progress Apps
I use the notes app on my smartphone to keep track of this. It's important that you're taking your measurements at the same time each week and that you only do it once a week, on the same day.

This gives you the most accurate results.

If you prefer specific apps to help with this, try the ones listed below:

1. **Simplenote App** - if you want to "write" your details down, this is a simplistic app that takes away all the fuss. I use this app to jot down what I did during my exercise session rather than taking down my measurements.
2. **Tracker - Fitness and Nutrition Tracking** - this app is great to not only track your workouts and weight/body fat, but you can also track your nutrition, which is great if you're struggling to stay on top of the food you're eating.
3. **Weight Loss Tracker** - this will purely track your weight and body fat, based on the information you provide. It's a nice, simple app for anyone that is looking to just track their

weight loss or keep an eye on their weight for maintenance purposes. iPhone and Android compatible.

4. **Fitlist - Workout & Fitness Tracker** - this is my favourite. You can enter in your own workouts and track your progress over time. iPhone and Android compatible.

I can't reiterate enough how important it is to keep track of your weight loss progress. Tracking and measuring are important to the success of your weight loss. Don't skip this step.

I have found that by sticking to just 30 minutes per day, 4 times a week, I am at my happiest.

Happy with the body I have and happy because I feel great! You can be the same to if you implement all you've learned inside this book.

The key is to start. Start slow and start small. Start with just 10 minutes a day and then build up to 30 minutes, then 60 minutes, whatever feels right for you.

I hope that I've been able to show you just how you can fit exercise into your day without joining the gym or owning equipment.

I hope you also realise that you have no excuse not to work out because everything in this book shows you that 30 minutes is all you need.

You also don't need weights, because you can stick to the body weight routines forever.

No excuses my friend.

Now, go forth and conquer... or just get your butt dressed in some workout gear and start!

CHAPTER 5: WHAT'S NEXT?

Next Steps

You've reached the end of the book and you've started your exercise regime... now you're ready to know what you should be doing next.

Don't forget to access the resources page to get access to even more resources and videos.

Visit this page: https:// www.hustleandgroove.com/ngnbresources

Password: ngnb@2717

And don't forget to grab your **Detox Your Diet Action Guide** here:
https://www.hustleandgroove.com/dydguide

Ok, so what's next?

Create Your Own Personalized Workouts

Creating your own workouts and exercise program is a great way to completely tailor an exercise routine to your specific needs.

Make sure that you always include cardio (when you can) and strength training in your workouts, as cardio alone won't provide your muscles with the resilience they need to support your body as you get older.

Steps to Create Your Personalized Workouts
Before you start creating your own workout, it's important to note that there is no 'one size fits all' when it comes to the steps outlined below.

During the exercises in this book, you should have figured out what works best for you. Remember this and you'll be fine.

And if at any point this just seems too hard, go back to basics and focus on the routines provided in this book.

1. Shoot for full body workouts - they are the easiest and unless you love doing weighted exercises or are really experienced, it's best to stick to body weight options for now
2. The areas below are what you should be working on when doing a full body workout:
    - Your quads (front of your legs)
    - Butt and hamstrings (back of your legs)
    - Chest, shoulders and triceps (push muscles)
    - Back, biceps and forearms (pull muscles)
    - Core (your abs and lower back)

Below are a list of exercises that target these areas.

To create your own routine, choose one exercise from each category and repeat each exercise 8-15 times, for

3-5 sets.

**_These should only be attempted once you've
completed at least 3 months of consistent exercise
using the routines in Chapter 4._**

Add in 10-15 minutes of cardio to round out each routine. You'll see cardio options below as well.

Quad Exercises:
- Squats
- Lunges
- One legged squats

Butt and Hamstring Exercises:
- Step ups
- Hip raises
- Glute bridges

Chest, Shoulders and Tricep Exercises:
- Overhead press
- Push-ups
- Dips

Back, Bicep and Forearm Exercises:
- Pull ups
- Inverse bodyweight rows

Core Exercises:
- Plank
- Side plank
- Mountain climbers

Cardio Options:
- Jumping jacks
- Jump rope
- Running (either on the spot or outside)
- High knees
- Jog in place
- Fast-paced walking

The art to creating a workout that you won't get bored with is to change it every 2-3 months.

Make sure that you allow 48 hours recovery time between each workout so that your muscles have time to recoup and so that you don't do yourself any injury.

Here's a sample program to kick your own ideas off.

Body-weight Workout:
Day 1 - Monday
Quads: 15 squats
Butt & Hamstrings: 15 hip raises
Chest, Shoulders & Triceps: 15 push-ups
Back, Biceps & Forearms: 15 bodyweight rows
Core: 30 second plank

Repeat 4 times (4 sets of each exercise).

Cardio: 10 minutes
:60 second jumping jacks
:60 second high knees
:60 second run in place

:60 second jump rope
:60 jog in place
:60 second jumping jacks
:60 second high knees
:60 second run in place
:60 second jump rope
:60 jog in place

Day 2 - Wednesday
Quads: 15 lunges
Butt & Hamstrings: 15 step ups
Chest, Shoulders & Triceps: 15 dips
Back, Biceps & Forearms: 15 push-ups
Core: 15 mountain climbers

Repeat 4 times (4 sets of each exercise).

Cardio: 10 minutes
:60 second jumping jacks
:60 second high knees
:60 second run in place
:60 second jump rope
:60 jog in place
:60 second jumping jacks
:60 second high knees
:60 second run in place
:60 second jump rope
:60 jog in place

Day 3 - Friday
Quads: 15 one-legged squats (each leg)
Butt & Hamstrings: 15 hip raises

Chest, Shoulders & Triceps: 15 push-ups
Back, Biceps & Forearms: 15 bodyweight rows
Core: 15 mountain climbers

Repeat 4 times (4 sets of each exercise).

Cardio: 10 minutes
:60 second jumping jacks
:60 second high knees
:60 second run in place
:60 second jump rope
:60 jog in place
:60 second jumping jacks
:60 second high knees
:60 second run in place
:60 second jump rope
:60 jog in place

Day 4 - Sunday
Quads: 15 walking lunges
Butt & Hamstrings: 15 hip raises
Chest, Shoulders & Triceps: 15 push-ups
Back, Biceps & Forearms: 15 bodyweight rows
Core: 30 second side plank (each side)

Repeat 4 times (4 sets of each exercise).

Cardio: 10 minutes
:60 second jumping jacks
:60 second high knees
:60 second run in place
:60 second jump rope

:60 jog in place
:60 second jumping jacks
:60 second high knees
:60 second run in place
:60 second jump rope
:60 jog in place

Remember, you can also refer to any of the workouts in this book to create your own program, and make sure that you know how to do each exercise properly.

If you want to make them harder, add weights to the exercises. Either household items, such as those mentioned throughout Chapter 4 or you can opt to purchase dumbbells or kettle bells, but these are definitely not necessary.

Listen to your body, if you find it difficult to do any of the exercises, reduce the amount of reps you're doing, making sure to increase them by 2-3 times the next time you attempt the exercise.

Want More?

If you want to feel good from the inside out, then my other book, *Detox Your Diet*, will help you figure out which foods don't gel with your body and what you can do to change this.

You will be guaranteed to lose 10-20 pounds in the first month following the steps outlined in this book!

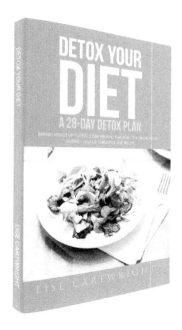

You can grab the book here: https://
www.detoxyourdietplan.com/the-book/

URGENT: CAN YOU HELP?

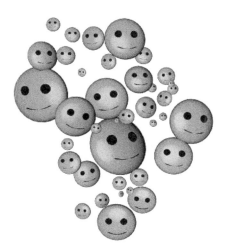

Thanks so much for downloading my book. I really appreciate your feedback and I LOVE hearing what you have to say.

If you enjoyed this book (even if you didn't), I'd love it if you left your **honest review on Amazon** by visiting this page:

Thanks so much!!

~ Lise

ABOUT THE AUTHOR

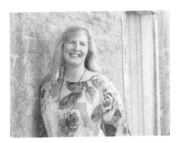

Lise Cartwright

Lise is an author, blogger and coach and a self-confessed shoe fanatic – she really is obsessed. Just ask her husband!

She has been looking for the magic in life since she was first exposed to positive, happy thoughts at the tender age of one - thanks Mum and Dad!

Lise can regularly be found at local cafes, drinking the more sophisticated and magical beverage that is a *Chai Latte*.

If you're looking to connect with Lise, you can stalk her on Facebook, tweet her on Twitter or send her an email.

Her online home is located at hustleandgroove.com.

Made in the USA
Monee, IL
26 June 2022

98636301R00046